How to handle Type 1 and Type 2 diabetes.

Mastering diabetes: prevent, handle, and manage.

By Linda J. Franklin

Table of content

Chapter 1: Recognizing the fundamentals.

Recognizing the fundamentals.

Diabetes Mellitus, or "diabetes," is a dangerous condition that develops when your body struggles to control the level of dissolved sugar (glucose) in your blood. It has nothing to do with the illness with the same name, Diabetes Insipidus, which causes issues with fluid retention in the kidneys.

Understanding the function that glucose performs in the body and what might occur when glucose control fails and blood sugar levels spike or fall dangerously low are prerequisites for understanding diabetes.

The organs, organelles, and cells that comprise the human body are living creatures that need sustenance to survive. Glucose is the sort of sugar that is used by cells. The body's cells, which are fixed in place, rely entirely on the bloodstream in which they are bathed to provide glucose to them. The body's cells quickly perish without enough glucose since they have no way to feed themselves.

People consume food, not glucose. As part of regular digestion, human meals are transformed into glucose. Upon conversion, glucose is released into the blood, increasing the blood's concentration of dissolved glucose. The body's tissues and cells get the dissolved glucose via the bloodstream.

Although there may be glucose in the blood, it cannot reach neighboring cells without the help of a chemical hormone called insulin. The cells can take in and use the glucose that is accessible because insulin works as a key to unlock the cells. In the presence of insulin, cells take up glucose from the blood, causing a decrease in blood sugar levels as the sugar leaves the circulation and enters the cells. Glucose may be thought of as being transported by insulin from the bloodstream to the cells. It's critical to comprehend that when insulin levels rise, blood sugar levels fall (because the sugar goes into the cells to be used for energy).

To maintain a constant supply of glucose in the blood to satisfy cell demands, the body is built to control and buffer the quantity of glucose dissolved in the blood. One of the numerous organs in your body, the pancreas, manufactures, stores, and releases insulin into circulation to lower blood sugar levels.

The quantity and kind of food that individuals consume affects the concentration of glucose that is readily accessible in the bloodstream at any one time. It is simple to convert refined carbs, candies, and sweets into glucose. Consequently, blood glucose levels quickly increase after consuming such items. In contrast, consuming more complex, unprocessed carbs (such as oatmeal, apples, baked potatoes, etc.) causes blood sugar levels to increase gradually and gradually because they take longer to digest and produce glucose. To prevent the deadly condition known as Hyperglycemia (high blood sugar), which will be discussed below, the body must respond swiftly by releasing huge quantities of insulin all at once in response to rapidly increase blood glucose concentrations.

As more insulin enters the system, glucose concentrations decrease as cells can use it. Unlike insulin levels, which fluctuate far more slowly, glucose levels may increase and decrease quickly. When a lot of simple sugar is consumed, glucose levels in the bloodstream rise fast. The pancreas releases insulin in reaction to the elevated sugar level. While the high amounts of insulin stay in circulation for a while, the glucose penetrates the cells quickly. An excess of insulin in the blood may arise from this, which may cause sensations of hunger and possibly hypoglycemia (low blood sugar), a severe disease. Less drastic correction is required when blood glucose levels increase more gradually. It is possible to release insulin in a safer, more regulated way that puts less pressure on the body. You will experience "fullness" or contentment for a longer length of time thanks to this more progressive procedure. Because of these factors, your general health should reduce the intake of sweets and processed sugars. Consume more complex sugars instead, such as those found in fresh fruit, whole wheat bread and pasta, and legumes. The distinction between white (simple) and whole wheat (more complex) bread serves as an example of the difference between simple and complex sugars (carbohydrates).

The capacity of the cell to utilize glucose depends on insulin. The body's delicately controlled glucose metabolism system may rapidly spiral out of control if there are issues with insulin production or with how insulin is perceived by the cells. When one or both of these issues arises, Diabetes sets in, blood sugar levels spike and fall, and the body is in danger of being harmed.

Chapter 2: Causes and types of diabetes

Understanding how the body typically uses glucose is essential to understanding diabetes.

How insulin works

Located below and behind the stomach, a gland produces the hormone insulin (pancreas).

Insulin is released by the pancreas into the blood.

Sugar can enter the cells as a result of insulin circulation.

The blood sugar level is decreased by insulin.

Insulin is secreted from the pancreas at a slower rate as blood sugar levels fall.

The function of glucose

The cells that makeup muscles and other tissues use glucose, a sugar, as a source of energy.

There are two main sources of glucose: food and the liver.

After being absorbed into the bloodstream, sugar uses insulin to enter cells.

The liver both produces and stores glucose.

When blood glucose levels are low, as they are when you haven't eaten in a while, the liver converts stored glycogen to glucose. Your glucose level is kept within a normal range as a result.

The majority of diabetes types lack a known precise cause. In every situation, blood sugar levels rise. This is due to insufficient insulin production by the pancreas. Combinations of genetic and environmental factors may contribute to the development of type 1 and type 2 diabetes. What those elements might be is unclear.

How diabetes affects blood sugar levels

The type of diabetes affects the risk factors. All types could be influenced by family history. The risk of type 1 diabetes can be increased by geographic factors and environmental factors.

The presence of diabetes immune system cells in family members of type 1 diabetics is occasionally tested (autoantibodies). You are more likely to develop type 1 diabetes if you have these autoantibodies. However, not everybody with these autoantibodies goes on to develop diabetes.

Your risk of developing type 2 diabetes may also be increased by your race or ethnicity. Certain people, including those who are Black, Hispanic, American Indian, and Asian American, are at a higher risk, though it is unclear why.

People who are overweight or obese are more likely to develop prediabetes, type 2 diabetes, and gestational diabetes.

Complications
Diabetes long-term complications appear over time. The risk of complications increases with the length of time you have diabetes and the degree of blood sugar control you maintain. Diabetes complications could eventually become fatal or even incapacitating. Indeed, type 2 diabetes can develop from prediabetes. Among the potential issues:

The disease of the heart and blood vessels (cardiovascular). The risk of many heart conditions is significantly increased by diabetes. These include heart attacks, strokes, arterial narrowing, and coronary artery disease with chest discomfort (angina) (atherosclerosis). Heart disease and stroke are more likely to occur if you have diabetes.

nerve injury (neuropathy). When consumed in excess, sugar can damage the capillary walls that feed the nerves, especially in the legs. When this happens, tingling, numbness, burning, or pain may result. Typically, these symptoms start at the tips of the toes or fingers and gradually move upward.

Digestion-related nerve damage can result in issues with nausea, vomiting, diarrhea, or constipation. Erectile dysfunction in men could result from it.

damaged kidneys (nephropathy). The kidneys contain millions of glomeruli, which are tiny blood vessel clusters that filter waste from the blood. This sensitive filtration system may be harmed by diabetes.

vision loss (retinopathy). Diabetes can harm the eye's blood vessels (diabetic retinopathy). The result could be blindness.

Foot damage Numerous foot complications are made more likely by nerve damage in the feet or poor blood circulation to the feet.

diseases of the mouth and skin. You may be more susceptible to bacterial and fungal infections on your skin if you have diabetes.

Deficiency in hearing. Diabetes patients experience hearing issues more frequently.

Alzheimer's illness Dementia, including Alzheimer's disease, may be more likely in people with type 2 diabetes.

Depression. Both type 1 and type 2 diabetics frequently experience depressive symptoms.

pregnancy-related diabetes complications

Most pregnant women with gestational diabetes have healthy babies. Blood sugar issues, however, can be problematic for both you and your unborn child if untreated or uncontrolled.

Gestational diabetes can result in several complications in your baby, including:

abnormal growth The placenta can allow for extra glucose. An increase in glucose causes the baby's pancreas to produce more insulin. As a result, your baby might become too big. It might necessitate a C-section occasionally and make labor challenges.

low sugar levels. After birth, babies of gestational diabetic mothers occasionally experience hypoglycemia or low blood sugar. This is a result of their high insulin production.

The later-life onset of type 2 diabetes. Babies whose mothers have gestational diabetes are more likely to grow up obese and develop type 2 diabetes.

Death. An unborn child's death before or soon after birth can result from untreated gestational diabetes.

Gestational diabetes can also result in complications in the mother, such as:

Preeclampsia. The signs of this condition include high blood pressure, excessive protein in the urine, and swelling in the legs and feet.
diabetes during pregnancy. If you previously experienced gestational diabetes, you are more likely to experience it again during your subsequent pregnancies.

Diabetic amputation and
Diabetes and bone and joint issues Show more relevant information
Prevention
There is no way to stop type 1 diabetes. However, the same healthy lifestyle decisions that help treat gestational diabetes, type 2 diabetes, and prediabetes can also help prevent them:

Consume healthy foods. Pick foods that are higher in fiber and lower in calories and fat.

Emphasize whole grains, fruits, and vegetables. Eat a variety of foods to avoid getting bored.

Increase your physical activity. On most days of the week, make an effort to engage in 30 minutes of moderate aerobic activity. Or try to complete at least 150 minutes of brisk aerobic exercise each week. For instance, go for a brisk daily walk. Break a long workout up into shorter sessions spread out throughout the day if you are unable to fit one in.

Reduce your weight. Diabetes risk can be lowered if you are overweight by losing even 7% of your body weight. Losing 14 pounds (6.4 kilograms), for instance, can reduce your risk of developing diabetes if you weigh 200 pounds (90.7 kilograms).

But avoid attempting to lose weight while expecting. How much weight you should gain during pregnancy is something you should discuss with your doctor.

Work on making long-term changes to your eating and exercise routines to keep your weight within a healthy range. A healthier heart, more energy, and improved self-esteem are just a few advantages of losing weight that you should keep in mind.

Drugs are a possibility on occasion. Metformin (Glumetza, Fortamet, and other brands) and other oral diabetes medications may reduce the risk of type 2 diabetes. But making good lifestyle choices is crucial. To be sure you haven't acquired type 2 diabetes if you have prediabetes, get your blood sugar tested at least once a year.

Treatment

As part of your doctor's prescribed regimen of medications, exercise, and dietary changes, you must closely monitor your blood sugar levels to keep them at a target level. The "seesaw effect" of rapidly fluctuating blood sugar levels, which may necessitate quick adjustments in medication dosages, particularly insulin, can be minimized or avoided by being mindful of what and when you eat. Learn how to pick the ideal diabetes treatment for you.

prescription medications for diabetes
The insulin that your body needs to utilize blood sugar for energy is no longer produced by your pancreas if you have type 1 diabetes. Injections of insulin or usage of a continuous pump will be necessary. Although learning how to administer injections to yourself, your infant, or your child may initially seem like the most difficult aspect of managing diabetes, it is much simpler than you might imagine.

Some diabetics use an automated pump known as an "insulin pump" that releases insulin on a predetermined schedule. The pump is configured by your doctor and you deliver a specific amount of insulin throughout the day (the basal dose). Additionally, you set the insulin pump to give a certain quantity of insulin depending on your blood sugar level before eating (bolus dose).

Five varieties of injectable insulin are available:
Rapid-acting (taking effect within a few minutes and lasting 2-4 hours)
Regular or momentary (taking effect within 30 minutes and lasting 3-6 hours)
Intermediate-acting (taking effect in 1-2 hours and lasting up to 18 hours)
Long-acting (taking effect in 1-2 hours and lasting beyond 24 hours)

Ultra-long-acting (taking effect in 1-2 hours and lasting 42 hours)

Additionally FDA-approved for use before meals are Afrezza, a rapid-acting inhaled insulin. It must be used in conjunction with long-acting insulin in type 1 diabetic patients; it should not be used by smokers or anyone with chronic lung disease. A single dosage cartridge is included. For those who need the use of many types of insulin, premixed insulin is also an option.

A basal dose of insulin that lasts for more than 42 hours is provided by the once-daily, long-acting insulin degludec (Tresiba). It is the only basal insulin that has been authorized for use in individuals with type 1 and types 2 diabetes who are as young as one year old. Rapid-acting insulin and it are combined to form Ryzodeg 70/30.

Each treatment program is personalized for the individual and may be changed according to the person's diet, level of activity, and reactions to stress and sickness.

Medicine for Diabetes

You can monitor your blood sugar levels, keep track of how much insulin your body requires as it changes, and collaborate with your doctor to determine the ideal insulin dose. Using a device known as a glucometer, diabetics may check their blood sugar up to many times each day. A little amount of your blood is dabbed on a strip of a special paper, and the glucometer counts the amount of glucose in the blood. Additionally, you may now connect continuous glucose monitoring systems (CGMS) to your body to monitor your blood sugar levels for up to a week at a time every few minutes. However, these devices are less accurate than a conventional glucometer and check blood glucose levels rather from the skin than from the blood.

Diet and exercise are sufficient for some type 2 diabetics to maintain disease management. Drugs like insulin and oral medications are necessary for some patients.

Different types of medications for type 2 diabetes help to return blood sugar levels to normal. They comprise:

Several medications, such as chlorpropamide (Diabinese), glimepiride (Amaryl), glipizide (Glucotrol), glyburide (DiaBeta, Glynase), nateglinide (Starlix), and repaglinide, boost the pancreas' secretion of insulin (Prandin)

Acarbose (Precose) and miglitol are two medications that prevent the intestines from absorbing sugar (Glyset)

Pioglitazone (Actos) and rosiglitazone, are two medications that enhance the body's use of insulin (Avandia)

Metformin is one example of a medication that reduces the liver's synthesis of sugar and improves insulin resistance (Glucophage). One method by which metformin helps restore normal blood sugar levels is by causing weight reduction.

Alogliptin (Nesina), dulaglutide (Trulicity), exenatide (Byetta, Bydureon), linagliptin (Tradjenta), liraglutide (Victoza), lixisenatide (Adlyxin), saxagliptin (Onglyza), semaglutide (Ozempic), and sitagliptin are some examples of medications that raise the pan (Januvia).

The sodium-glucose co-transporter 2 (SGLT2) inhibitors are medications that prevent the kidneys from reabsorbing glucose and increase the amount of glucose excreted in the urine. They also cause weight reduction, which aids in returning blood sugar levels to normal. They are the following: ertugliflozin, empagliflozin, dapagliflozin, and canagliflozin (Invokana, Farxiga) (Steglatro). Additionally, these medications may aid heart failure patients in lowering their risk of cardiovascular mortality and heart failure-related hospitalization.

A synthetic hormone for injection is called pramlintide (Symlin). In diabetics who take insulin, it helps reduce blood sugar levels after meals.

Multiple diabetic medications may be included in certain tablets. They consist of the newly authorized linagliptin/epagliflozin combination (Glyxambi). It combines a DPP-4 inhibitor, which raises hormone production, with an SGLT2 inhibitor, which prevents the kidneys from reabsorbing glucose.

Chapter 3: Type 2 diabetes

A lifelong condition, type 2 diabetes prevents your body from properly using insulin. Insulin resistance is a condition that affects people with type 2 diabetes.

The majority of those who develop this type of diabetes are middle-aged or older people. It was formerly known as adult-onset diabetes. However, type 2 diabetes also affects children and adolescents, largely as a result of childhood obesity.

The most typical type of diabetes is type 2. There are about 29 million types 2 diabetics in the United States. Another 84 million people have prediabetes, which is high blood sugar (or blood glucose) but not quite high enough to be classified as diabetes.

Type 2 Diabetes Symptoms and Signs
You might not even notice type 2 diabetes symptoms if they are only mild. There are

about 8 million people who have it but are unaware of it. Some signs are:

having a lot of thirsts
many urination
cloudy vision
being grumpy
Numbness or tingling in your hands or feet
Feeling worn out or fatigued
Non-healing injuries
yeast infections that recur frequently
feeling peckish
Loss of weight without effort
Increased infection rate
Consult a physician if you notice any dark rashes under your arms or around your neck. These are referred to as acanthosis nigricans, and they might indicate that your body is starting to become insulin resistant.

Diabetes Type 2 Causes
Insulin is a hormone that is produced in your pancreas. It aids in the conversion of glucose, a type of sugar from the food you

eat, into energy in your cells. Type 2 diabetics produce insulin, but their cells don't use it as effectively as they should.

To try to get glucose into your cells, your pancreas initially produces more insulin. The glucose builds up in your blood as a result when it eventually can't keep up.

Type 2 diabetes is typically brought on by several factors. They could consist of:

Genes. Different DNA snippets that influence how your body produces insulin have been discovered by scientists.
additional mass. In particular, if you carry your extra weight around your midsection, being overweight or obese can lead to insulin resistance.
Syndrome metabolic. High blood sugar, excess belly fat, high blood pressure, high cholesterol, and high triglycerides are a few of the conditions that people with insulin resistance frequently experience.

excessive liver glucose production When you have low blood sugar, your liver produces and releases glucose. Your blood sugar increases after eating, and typically your liver slows down and stores its glucose for later. However, not everyone's livers do. They continue producing sugar.

poor cell-to-cell communication Cells can occasionally send incorrect signals or misinterpret messages. Diabetes can develop as a result of a series of issues that affect how your cells produce and utilize insulin or glucose.

damaged beta cells. Your blood sugar levels fluctuate if the insulin-producing cells release the incorrect amount of insulin at the incorrect time. These cells may also suffer harm from high blood sugar.

Risk factors for diabetes
You're more likely to develop type 2 diabetes if certain factors exist. Your likelihood of

receiving it increases as more of these apply to you. Certain factors are connected to who you are:

45 years or older
Family. a brother, sister, or parent with diabetes
Ethnicity. Asian, Hispanic, Native American, Alaska Native, Native American, Pacific Islander, or African American
Your medical history and current state of health are risk factors as well as:

Prediabetes
vascular and cardiovascular disease
even when managed and treated, high blood pressure
low levels of good cholesterol (HDL)
elevated triglycerides
being obese or overweight
having a child who was over 9 pounds
gestational diabetes during pregnancy
Ovarian polycystic disease (PCOS)
Depression

Your daily routine and lifestyle are also factors that increase your risk of developing diabetes. You can take action against the following:

exercising insufficiently or not at all
Smoking\sStress
excessive or insufficient sleep
Diagnosis and Tests for Type 2 Diabetes
Blood tests by your doctor can check for type 2 diabetes symptoms. To confirm the diagnosis, they typically test you twice a day. However, one test might be sufficient if your blood sugar is extremely high or you have numerous symptoms.

A1c. It resembles an average of your blood glucose levels over the previous two to three months.
fasting blood sugar. It's also referred to as a fasting blood sugar test. On an empty stomach, it checks your blood sugar. For eight hours before the test, you are only permitted to consume water.

oral test for glucose tolerance (OGTT). To determine how your body reacts to the sugar, check your blood sugar before and two hours after consuming something sweet.

Treatment for Type 2 Diabetes

A combination of lifestyle modifications and medication is used to manage type 2 diabetes.

changes in lifestyle

You might be able to control your blood sugar levels only through diet and exercise.

losing weight Losing extra weight can help. While losing 5% of your body weight is beneficial, losing at least 7% of it and maintaining it seems ideal. Therefore, losing about 13 pounds can lower blood sugar levels in a person who weighs 180 pounds. Portion control and eating healthy foods are good places to start if you want to lose weight, even though they can seem overwhelming.

a nutritious diet. For type 2 diabetes, there is no special diet. You can learn about carbs from a registered dietitian, who can also assist you in creating a meal plan you can follow. Focus on:

consuming less energy

Cutting down on refined carbohydrates, particularly sweets

Including fruits and vegetables in your diet

Increased fiber intake

Exercise. Try to engage in physical activity for 30 to 60 minutes each day. Exercises that raise your heart rate include walking, biking, swimming, and other activities. Combine that with strength training exercises like weightlifting or yoga. You might require a snack before exercise if you take a medication that lowers your blood sugar.

Keep an eye on your blood sugar levels. Your doctor will advise you as to whether you should test your blood sugar levels and how often to do so, depending on your therapy, particularly if you are using insulin.

Medication

You could require medication if changing your way of life doesn't help you reach your goal blood sugar levels. The most frequent signs of type 2 diabetes include:

Metformin (Fortamet, Glucophage, Glumetza, Riomet) (Fortamet, Glucophage, Glumetza, Riomet). Usually, type 2 diabetes is treated with this as the first medication. It lessens the amount of glucose your liver produces and enhances the effectiveness of the insulin your liver does produce.
Sulfonylureas. These medicines encourage your body to produce more insulin. Glyburide, glimepiride (Amaryl), and glipizide (Glucotrol, Metaglip) are a few of them (DiaBeta, Micronase).

Meglitinides. They work more quickly than sulfonylureas and aid in the production of more insulin by your body. Take nateglinide (Starlix) or repaglinide, as necessary (Prandin).

Thiazolidinediones. They increase your insulin sensitivity, much like metformin does. Pioglitazone (Actos) or rosiglitazone are two options (Avandia). However, they also increase your risk of developing heart issues, so they aren't typically the first course of treatment.

DPP-4 repressants. These drugs, linagliptin (Tradjenta), saxagliptin (Onglyza), and sitagliptin (Januvia), help lower blood sugar levels, but they can also cause joint pain and possibly aggravate pancreatic inflammation.

GLP-1 receptor agonists To slow digestion and lower blood sugar levels, you administer these medications with a needle. They include exenatide (Byetta, Bydureon), liraglutide (Victoza), and semaglutide (Ozempic).

inhibitors of SGLT2. Your kidneys can remove more glucose thanks to these. You could receive empagliflozin, dapagliflozin, or canagliflozin (Invokana, Farxiga) (Jardiance). The risk of hospitalization or death from heart failure has also been shown to be significantly lower when empagliflozin is used.

agonist for GIP and GLP-1 receptors. The GLP-1 and GIP receptors are both activated by tirzepatide (Mounjaro), the first drug of its kind, which results in better blood sugar regulation.

Insulin. You could inject yourself with long-lasting medications like insulin detemir (Levemir) or insulin glargine at night (Lantus).

Your blood sugar may gradually worsen even if you alter your lifestyle and take your medication as prescribed. That in no way implies that you did anything wrong. Diabetes is a progressive condition, and many people eventually require multiple medications.

Combination therapy is the term used when more than one medication is used to manage type 2 diabetes.

Symptoms of Type 2 Diabetes
Type 2 Diabetes Treatment Glucose Test for Diabetes
To determine the right combination for you, you and your doctor should collaborate. You usually continue taking metformin and add another medication.

Depending on your position, that may be anything. For instance, some medications manage blood sugar spikes that occur immediately after meals (your doctor may refer to this condition as hyperglycemia). Hypoglycemia, or blood sugar drops between meals, can be prevented more successfully by others. Along with your diabetes, some may aid in weight loss or lowering cholesterol.

Discuss any potential side effects with your doctor. The cost could be a problem as well.

Any decision you make will need to take into account whether you also take medication for another condition.

When you begin taking a new drug combination, you'll require more frequent visits to the doctor.

You might discover that taking a second medication isn't enough to control your blood sugar. Or the two medications combined might only be effective temporarily. If that occurs, your doctor might suggest a third non-insulin medication or start you on insulin therapy.

Diabetes Type 2 Prevention
You can reduce your risk of developing diabetes by leading a healthy lifestyle.

Lose weight. Your risk of type 2 diabetes can be reduced by half with just a 7% to 10% weight loss.

Start moving. You can reduce your risk by almost a third by walking briskly for 30 minutes each day.

Wholesome eating Trans and saturated fats, as well as excessively processed carbohydrates, should be avoided. Limit red and processed meats.

Stop smoking. To avoid creating a new issue by addressing an existing one, see your doctor about how to avoid gaining weight after quitting.

Complications of Type 2 Diabetes

Over time, elevated blood sugar may harm and interfere with:

circulatory system and heart. Heart disease and stroke risk are increased by up to five times. Atherosclerosis-related blood vessel blockages and chest discomfort are also quite likely to occur to you (angina).

Kidneys. You could need dialysis or a kidney transplant if your kidneys are damaged or failing.

Eyes. The little blood vessels in your eyes' backs might get damaged by high blood sugar (retinopathy). Blindness may result from this if it is not addressed.

Nerves. This may affect your ability to digest food, your ability to feel your feet, and how you react sexually.

Skin. Because your blood doesn't circulate as effectively, wounds heal more slowly and are more likely to get an infection.

Pregnancy. Women who have diabetes are more likely to have miscarriages, stillbirths, or give birth to a child who has a birth defect.

Sleep. Your breathing may stop and resume while you sleep, a condition known as sleep apnea.

Hearing. It's not quite apparent why you have a higher likelihood of having hearing issues.

Brain. High blood sugar levels may harm your brain and increase your chances of developing Alzheimer's disease.

Depression. Those who have the illness are twice as likely to experience depression as those who do not.

Maintaining good control of your type 2 diabetes is the best strategy to prevent these consequences.

Remember to take your insulin or diabetic meds on schedule.

Check your blood sugar.

Don't miss meals and follow a healthy diet.

To check for early warning signs of problems, visit your doctor frequently.

Chapter 4:Diet to eat and avoid.

Fattening

Omega-3 fatty acids DHA and EPA, which have significant advantages for heart health, are found in abundance in fish including salmon, sardines, herring, anchovies, and mackerel.

For those with diabetes, who have a higher risk of heart disease and stroke, it's crucial to regularly consume enough of these fats.

DHA and EPA guard the cells that line your blood vessels, lower inflammation-related signs, and could even help your arteries work better.

According to research, those who consume fatty fish regularly are less likely to get acute coronary syndromes, such as heart attacks, and to pass away from heart disease (2).

Consuming fatty fish may also help control blood sugar, according to studies.

According to research involving 68 overweight or obese people, those who ingested fatty fish saw substantial reductions in post-meal blood sugar levels compared to those who received lean fish.

Additionally, fish is a fantastic source of high-quality protein, which keeps you full and helps to control blood sugar levels.
Omega-3 fats, which are found in fatty fish, may help lower inflammation and other risk factors for heart disease and stroke. Furthermore, it's a fantastic source of protein, which is crucial for controlling blood sugar.

Leafy greens
Leafy green vegetables are very calorie-efficient and nutrient-dense.

They don't substantially alter blood sugar levels since they contain relatively little digestible carbohydrates or carbs that the body can absorb.

Many vitamins and minerals, including vitamin C, are abundant in spinach, kale, and other leafy greens.
According to some data, persons with diabetes have lower vitamin C levels than those without the disease, and they could also need more vitamin C overall.
Both an effective antioxidant and an anti-inflammatory, vitamin C is.

People with diabetes may boost their blood vitamin C levels and decrease inflammation and cellular damage by increasing their dietary consumption of foods high in vitamin C.

Leafy green veggies are full of vitamins and minerals including vitamin C and antioxidants that are good for your eyes and heart health.

(3) Avocados
You don't need to be concerned about avocados raising your blood sugar levels since they contain less than 1 gram of sugar, little carbs, a lot of fiber, and beneficial fats.

Consuming avocados is also linked to a better quality diet overall, as well as significantly lower body weight and BMI.
This makes avocados the perfect food for diabetics, particularly given that obesity raises the risk of acquiring diabetes.

Avocados might offer special diabetes-prevention-related qualities.
A lipid molecule called avocatin B (AvoB), which is uniquely present in avocados, has been shown in a 2019 mouse research to suppress incomplete oxidation in skeletal muscle and the pancreas, hence lowering insulin resistance.

Establishing the link between avocados and the prevention of diabetes will need further human study.

Avocados are linked to better overall diet quality and contain less than 1 gram of sugar. Avocados may possess qualities that are specifically suited to preventing diabetes.

4. Eggs

You may lower your risk of heart disease in several ways by regularly eating eggs.

Eggs may reduce inflammation, enhance insulin sensitivity, raise HDL levels (the good cholesterol), and alter the size and structure of LDL (the bad cholesterol).

Having eggs for breakfast might help diabetics control their blood sugar levels throughout the day, according to 2019 research. Eggs are heavy in fat and low in carbohydrates.

Consuming eggs has been related in earlier studies to heart problems in diabetics.
However, a more recent analysis of research indicated that eating 6–12 eggs per week as part of a healthy diet did not raise heart disease risk factors in those with diabetes.

Furthermore, some evidence indicates that consuming eggs may lower the risk of stroke.

Eggs may lower your risk of heart disease, support healthy blood sugar regulation, safeguard your eye health, and help you feel full.

Chia seeds, no. 5
People with diabetes should eat chia seeds often.
They have a very high fiber content but little carbohydrates that can be digested.

In reality, fiber, which doesn't boost blood sugar, makes up 11 of the 12 grams of carbohydrates in a 28-gram (1-ounce) meal of chia seeds.

Because food travels through your intestines more slowly and is digested more slowly, the viscous fiber in chia seeds may reduce your blood sugar levels.

Chia seeds may aid in maintaining a healthy weight since fiber curbs appetite and helps you feel full. Chia seeds may also support diabetics' glucose control.

Eating chia seeds boosts weight reduction and aids in maintaining excellent glycemic control, according to research including 77 persons with type 2 diabetes who were overweight or obese.

Chia seeds have also been shown to assist in lowering inflammatory indicators and blood pressure.

High fiber content can potentially aid in weight loss thanks to chia seeds. They also assist in preserving blood glucose levels.

6. Beans
Beans are very cheap, filling, and healthy.

A kind of legume known as beans is high in fiber, calcium, potassium, and other healthy minerals.

They have a very low glycemic index as well, which is crucial for controlling diabetes.
Diabetes prevention may also be aided by beans.

Higher consumption of legumes was associated with a lower risk of type 2 diabetes in a study involving more than 3,000 participants at high risk of cardiovascular disease.
Beans are a good choice for diabetics since they are affordable, filling, and have a low glycemic index.

Seven. Greek yogurt
Daily yogurt consumption was associated with an 18% decreased risk of type 2

diabetes, according to long-term research incorporating health information from more than 100,000 people (13 Trusted Source).

If losing weight is a personal objective of yours, it could also aid in that.
According to studies, type 2 diabetics who consume yogurt and other dairy products may experience weight reduction and an improvement in their body composition (14 Trusted Source).

Yogurt has significant quantities of protein, calcium, and a unique kind of fat called conjugated linoleic acid (CLA), which may help you feel fuller for longer.
Greek yogurt is also lower in carbohydrates than regular yogurt, with just 6 to 8 grams per cup.

It also contains more protein, which may help people lose weight by lowering their appetite and calorie consumption.

Yogurt may support normal blood sugar levels, lower heart disease risk factors, and aid with weight control.

8. Nuts

Nuts are tasty and wholesome.

Although some have more than others, most nut varieties are low in net carbohydrates and include fiber.

Research on a range of nuts has shown that frequent eating may decrease blood sugar, LDL (bad) cholesterol and HbA1c (a measure for long-term blood sugar control) levels as well as reduce inflammation.

Nuts may also assist diabetics to improve the condition of their hearts.

Eaten tree nuts, such as walnuts, almonds, hazelnuts, and pistachios, lessen the risk of heart disease and mortality, according to 2019 research including more than 16,000 people with type 2 diabetes (15Trusted Source).

Nuts may lower blood sugar levels, according to research.
According to type 2 diabetes research, regular use of walnut oil reduced blood sugar levels.
Because type 2 diabetics often have high insulin levels, which are connected to fat, this result is crucial.
Nuts are a nutritious supplement to a diet that is balanced. Due to their high fiber content, they may lower LDL (bad) cholesterol and blood sugar levels.

9. Broccoli Broccoli is one of the veggies with the highest nutritional value.
In addition to essential nutrients like vitamin C and magnesium, a half cup of cooked broccoli only has 27 calories and 3 grams of digestible carbohydrates.

Managing your blood sugar levels may also be aided by broccoli.

According to one study, eating broccoli sprouts caused diabetics' blood glucose levels to drop.

Sulforaphane, a substance found in cruciferous vegetables like broccoli and sprouts, is probably to blame for this drop in blood sugar levels.

Broccoli has a high nutrient content and is a low-calorie, low-carb food. It is bursting with beneficial plant substances that could offer defense against several diseases.

Olive oil extra virgin 10.

Oleic acid, monounsaturated fat found in extra-virgin olive oil, may help with glycemic control, lower fasting and post-meal triglyceride levels, and have antioxidant effects.

Because people with diabetes frequently struggle to control their blood sugar levels and have high triglyceride levels, this is crucial.

The satiation hormone GLP-1 may also be stimulated by oleic acid.

Olive oil was the only fat found in a thorough analysis of 32 studies looking at various types of fat to lower the risk of heart disease.

Polyphenols are another type of antioxidant found in olive oil.

Polyphenols lower blood pressure, protect the cells lining your blood vessels, prevent oxidation from harming your LDL (bad) cholesterol, and reduce inflammation.

Since extra-virgin olive oil hasn't been refined, it hasn't lost any of its beneficial antioxidants or other qualities.

Because many extra-virgin olive oils are blended with less expensive oils like corn and soy, be sure to select this type from a reputable supplier.

Beneficial oleic acid is found in extra-virgin olive oil. Blood pressure and heart health are both improved by it.
The flaxseeds
Flaxseeds also referred to as common flax or linseeds, are rich in fiber, special plant compounds, and heart-healthy omega-3 fats.
They contain lignans, which make up a portion of their insoluble fiber and may help lower the risk of heart disease and enhance blood sugar control.
A review of 25 randomized clinical trials revealed a significant link between whole flaxseed supplementation and lower blood sugar levels .

Blood pressure may be reduced by flax seeds as well.

A 2016 study with prediabetic participants found that consuming flaxseed powder daily decreased blood pressure, but did not improve glycemic control or insulin resistance.

Flaxseed's potential to prevent or manage diabetes requires further study.
However, flaxseed is generally good for your gut and heart health.

Furthermore, flaxseeds have a high viscous fiber content that enhances gut health, insulin sensitivity, and feelings of fullness.
Flaxseeds may assist in reducing inflammation, lowering the risk of heart disease, lowering blood sugar levels, and enhancing insulin sensitivity.

Vines and apple cider vinegar, 12.
Both apple cider vinegar and regular vinegar have numerous health advantages.
Despite being made from apples, acetic acid is produced through the fermentation of fruit sugar. Less than 1 gram of carbohydrates per tablespoon is present in the final product.

Vinegar lowers fasting blood sugar and HbA1c levels, according to a meta-analysis of six studies involving 317 people with type 2 diabetes.

Antimicrobial and antioxidant effects are just two of the many potential health benefits of apple cider vinegar. To confirm its health advantages, however, more research is required.

Start by adding 4 teaspoons of apple cider vinegar to a glass of water each day before each meal to incorporate it into your diet. To ensure that the taste is not too overpowering, consider adding 1 teaspoon per glass of water. A maximum of 4 tablespoons should be consumed each day.

Although more research is required to confirm apple cider vinegar's health advantages, it may help lower fasting blood sugar levels.

14. Strawberry
The anthocyanins, which give strawberries their red color, are powerful antioxidants.

In addition, they contain polyphenols, which are advantageous plant substances with antioxidant properties.
In adults with overweight and obesity who were not diabetic, a 2017 study found that consuming the polyphenols from strawberries and cranberries for six weeks increased insulin sensitivity.

Because low insulin sensitivity can result in excessively high blood sugar levels, this is crucial information.

About 53.1 calories and 12.7 grams of carbohydrates, including three fiber-rich grams, are present in a 1-cup serving of strawberries (24Trusted Source).

Along with providing more than 100% of the recommended daily intake (RDI) for vitamin C, this serving also has additional anti-inflammatory benefits for heart health.

SYNOPSIS Strawberries are a low-sugar fruit that is highly anti-inflammatory and may reduce insulin resistance.

15 Garlic

Garlic is surprisingly nutrient-dense for its diminutive size and low-calorie content.

Raw garlic contains about 4 calories in one clove or 3 grams.

Manganese: 2% of the daily value (DV)
A 2% daily value for vitamin B6
Vitamin C: 1 percent of the DV
Selenium: 1 percent of the DV
Fibre: 0.06 grams
Garlic, according to research, helps manage blood sugar levels and can control cholesterol (26Trusted Source).

Even though the meta-analysis cited above only included servings from 0.05 to 1.5 grams, many studies that conclude that garlic is a proven healthy option for people with diabetes include abnormal dietary amounts of garlic.

One garlic clove weighs approximately 3 grams for context.

Garlic has been shown in studies to lower blood pressure and control cholesterol levels.

In diabetics, garlic helps reduce blood sugar, inflammation, LDL cholesterol, and blood pressure.

15. Squash One of the healthiest vegetables available is the variety-rich squash.

The dense, filling food has a low glycemic index and has only a few calories per serving.

Acorn, pumpkin, and butternut are some winter varieties with a tough exterior.

The peel of summer squash is edible and soft. Zucchini and Italian squash are the most popular varieties.

Squash includes healthy antioxidants, like the majority of vegetables. In addition, squash has less sugar than sweet potatoes, making it a superior substitute.

Pumpkin polysaccharides, which are also present in squash, have been shown in studies to improve insulin tolerance and lower blood glucose levels in rats .

Squash reduced high blood glucose levels in diabetics who were critically ill quickly and effectively, according to a small human study, despite the paucity of human research in this area.

To confirm squash's health advantages, more human studies are required.

However, squash is a fantastic addition to any meal due to its many health advantages.

Winter and summer squash both have healthy antioxidants that may help lower blood sugar.

Shirataki ramen 16.

The benefits of shirataki noodles for managing diabetes and weight are numerous.

These noodles contain significant amounts of the konjac root fiber glucomannan.

Shirataki, a type of noodles or rice made from this plant, is produced in Japan.

Glucomannan is a form of viscous fiber, which makes you feel full and pleased.
It has also been demonstrated to lower blood sugar levels after meals and enhance heart disease risk factors in individuals with diabetes and metabolic syndrome (29Trusted Source).

One study found that glucomannan significantly lowered the fasting blood glucose, serum insulin, and cholesterol levels in diabetic rats.

Shirataki noodles are only 10 calories per serving and have just 3 grams of digestible carbs in a 3.5-ounce (100-gram) serving.
The noodles must, however, be thoroughly rinsed before use because they are frequently packaged with a liquid that smells fishy.

The noodles should then be cooked for a few minutes over high heat without any additional fat to achieve a texture that resembles that of noodles.

Shirataki noodles contain glucomannan, which can help with blood sugar control and cholesterol levels while promoting feelings of fullness.

meals to omit
Understanding which foods to limit is just as crucial to managing diabetes as knowing which foods to include.
This is due to the high carbohydrate and added sugar content of many foods and beverages, which can raise blood sugar levels. Other foods might have a detrimental effect on cardiovascular health or promote weight gain.

The following foods are ones you should limit or stay away from if you have diabetes.

Refined grains

Because refined grains lack fiber and are high in carbohydrates, they can cause blood sugar levels to rise more quickly than whole grains. Examples of refined grains include white bread, pasta, and rice.

One review of the literature found that whole grain rice, as opposed to white rice, was significantly more effective at regulating blood sugar levels after a meal (32Trusted Source).

2. beverages sweetened with sugar

Sugar-sweetened drinks like soda, sweet tea, and energy drinks not only lack essential nutrients, but each serving also contains a high concentration of sugar, which can raise blood sugar levels.

Foods that have been fried

Trans fat, a type of fat that has been connected to a higher risk of heart disease, is a common ingredient in fried foods.

Furthermore, the high-calorie content of fried foods like potato chips, french fries, and mozzarella sticks may help with weight gain.

Alcohol 4.
Alcohol consumption should be kept to a minimum for those with diabetes. This is due to the possibility of low blood sugar is increased by alcohol, especially if it is consumed on an empty stomach.
Five. Breakfast cereal
Most types of breakfast cereal contain a lot of added sugar. Some brands contain the same amount of sugar per serving as some desserts.
When buying cereal, be sure to carefully read the nutrition label and choose a variety that contains little sugar. Choose oatmeal instead, and add some fresh fruit to it to naturally sweeten it.

6. Candy

Each serving of candy has a lot of sugar in it. It typically has a high glycemic index, which means it's likely to result in blood sugar spikes and crashes after eating.

Processed meats

Cold cuts, bacon, hot dogs, salami, and other processed meats have high salt content as well as other unhealthy additives. Additionally, a higher risk of heart disease has been linked to eating processed meats.

A fruit juice 8.

If you have diabetes, it's preferable to stick to whole fruit whenever feasible, even if 100% fruit juice may be sometimes consumed in moderation.

Fruit juice lacks the fiber required to help balance blood sugar levels but has all the carbohydrates and sugar found in fresh fruit, which explains why.

MEDICAL RESOURCE

creating a strategy

Planning a balanced, healthful diet for diabetes may be done using several techniques.

using a plate

Without counting or measuring your meals, using the plate technique may help promote balanced blood sugar levels. To make a nutritionally balanced dinner, you must change the quantities of certain food categories on your plate.

Simply place non-starchy vegetables, such as leafy greens, broccoli, squash, or cauliflower, in the middle of your plate to begin.

Proteins like chicken, turkey, eggs, fish, tofu, and lean beef or pork should make up one-fourth of your meal.

A healthy source of carbs should be included on the remaining quarter of the plate, such as whole grains, legumes, starchy vegetables, fruit, or dairy products.

A low-calorie beverage, including water, unsweetened tea, black coffee, or club soda, should be had with your meal to help you keep hydrated.

Index glycomic

A useful tool for regulating blood sugar levels is the glycemic index. Based on their glycemic index, it classifies foods as having a high, low, or medium GI to indicate how much they raise blood sugar levels.

When using this approach, try to avoid foods with high glycemic indexes and instead restrict your consumption of those with low or medium glycemic indexes.

This article has further details on the glycemic index and how to utilize it to better regulate blood sugar levels.

Calorie counting

By keeping track of how many carbs you eat throughout the day, carb counting is a well-liked technique for controlling blood sugar levels.

Monitoring the grams of carbohydrates in the meals you consume is required. Depending on how many carbohydrates you ingest, you could sometimes also need to change the insulin dose.

Depending on your age, size, and degree of activity, as well as other variables, you should consume different amounts of carbohydrates at each meal and snack.

You may thus develop a personalized carb counting strategy depending on your requirements with the aid of a licensed dietitian or physician.

menu example

Healthy eating doesn't have to be challenging or time-consuming when you have diabetes.

Here is a one-day example menu with a few quick dinner suggestions to get you started:

Breakfast: an omelet with peppers, broccoli, and mushrooms

A handful of almonds for breakfast

Grilled chicken salad for lunch with spinach, tomatoes, avocado, onions, cucumber, and balsamic vinaigrette

Greek yogurt with sliced strawberries and walnuts makes a tasty afternoon snack.
Dinner will include baked salmon, quinoa, and asparagus.
Snack for later: sliced vegetables and hummus

Uncontrolled diabetes raises your chance of developing several severe illnesses.
However, consuming foods that support healthy levels of insulin, blood sugar, and inflammation may significantly lower your risk of problems.

Just keep in mind that although these meals may aid in blood sugar control, maintaining a generally nutrient-rich, balanced diet is the most crucial aspect of optimal blood sugar management.

Chapter 5:How to prevent diabetes

So, how can you prevent diabetes in your family and yourself? And if you have a diagnosis, what can you do? The good news is that you may significantly increase your chances of avoiding diabetes or guarding against its consequences by modifying certain lifestyle choices.

1. Keep a normal weight.
Obesity and type 2 diabetes have been associated directly. Fat may make the body's cells resistant to insulin, which might be one explanation for this. The foods that promote weight gain and obesity, such as processed foods rich in sugar, salt, and saturated fat, are also associated with the development of diabetes, particularly sugary beverages.

Start small while trying to reduce weight. Your health might benefit from losing even 10 to 15 pounds.

2. Adopt a balanced diet.

In addition to being beneficial for your general health and for helping you lose weight, a balanced diet is essential for avoiding and managing diabetes. The following should be part of your diet:

different fruits and veggies (frozen fruits and vegetables with no added fat or sugar are also excellent options)

Lean meats and fish

dairy without added fat

grainy foods

the good fats

Avoid eating fried food, processed food, sweet beverages and sweets, foods rich in salt, and foods high in trans and saturated fat.

Concentrate on eating modest, evenly spaced meals throughout the day to keep blood sugar levels in a normal range. Avoid missing meals since doing so might increase blood sugar levels and cause weight gain.

3. Move forward!
To live an active lifestyle, you don't need specialized gear or a pricey gym membership. Exercise may aid in weight loss and improve blood circulation, which is hampered by diabetes. Here are some ideas of physical activities you may start doing right now:

jogging in the neighborhood or close to the workplace
cleaning your residence
Gardening
cleaning your vehicle
Strength training (push-ups, squats, lunges, crunches, etc.)
In a public pool, doing laps
marching while watching TV or talking on the phone (or just pacing about)
Be imaginative with your activity! You're acting healthily as long as you're moving.

4. Give up smoking.

Your likelihood of acquiring cardiovascular disease is significantly increased by diabetes. Additionally, as smoking reduces blood flow and elevates blood pressure, it increases your risk of developing cardiovascular disease and stroke.

5. Take your medicine.
You must take your meds exactly as prescribed if you already have diabetes. Even those with a greater risk of developing the condition often get pharmaceutical recommendations from their physicians. Consult your doctor or pharmacist if you have any queries regarding your medicines.

6. Have your blood sugar checked.
If you have been given a diabetes diagnosis, your doctor could advise using a blood glucose meter to monitor your blood sugar. Your diabetes will be easier to manage with the aid of this meter. If you believe a glucose meter is the best option for you, talk to your doctor.

7. Obtain aid.

Do you or someone you care about have a diabetes risk? Does the illness currently have an impact on your life? Help is available from us.

Diabetes should be eradicated from the Southeast, according to Erlanger. To understand how you may live a diabetes-free life, speak with your primary care physician about your worries or schedule an appointment at one of our nearby health clinics.